Copyright ©

All rights reserved. No part of this publication maybe reproduced, distributed, or transmitted in any form or by any means, including photocopying, recording, or other electronic or mechanical methods, without the prior written permission of the publisher, except in the case of brief quotations embodied in critical reviews and certain other noncommercial uses permitted by copyright law.

Contents

Irritable bowel syndrome (IBS) 6

Symptoms 7

Causes 9

Is it curable? 11

Treatment 12

Diagnosis 17

Risk factors 20

IBS diet 22

Foods that may trigger IBS 25

Alternatives to trigger foods 28

The IBS seven-day eating plan 31

Tips for eating out 37

Other strategies 39

Outlook 40

IBD DIET RECIPES 41

Miso Braised Eggplant 41

Sticky sprout and celeriac mash 44

Coconut Candy 47

Greek Lamb Salad 51

Blueberry And Lemon Buttermilk Pancakes 54

Muesli 58

Kiwi Smoothie 61

Chocolate Chip-Oat Scones 63

COCONUT OAT GRANOLA WITH CHOCOLATE AND ROSEWATER CREAM 68

POACHED EGG WITH YOGURT AND GARLIC-INFUSED OIL 72

Quinoa Porridge with Berries 74

Spaghetti Bolognese 77

Maple Garlic Glazed Salmon 81

Bibimbap Nourishing Bowl 83

Chilli Coconut Crusted Fish with Salad 86

LASAGNA BOLOGNESE 91

Cheesy Baked Quinoa and Zucchini Cups 95

Banana Nut Quinoa Muffins 96

Kettle Popcorn Recipe; Gluten-free, Vegan 99

Homemade Trail mix 101

Chewy Peanut Butter Cookies 102

Blueberry Crumble Slice 104

Fudgy One-Bowl Brownies 109

Creamy Coconut Milk Quinoa Pudding 113

FERRERO ROCHER 115

SOMMER'S STROGANOFF 117

Baked French Toast 121

PALEO & LOW FODMAP SWEET AND SOUR CHICKEN 125

Irritable bowel syndrome (IBS)

Irritable bowel syndrome (IBS) is a long term gastrointestinal disorder that can cause persistent discomfort. However, most people will not experience severe complications.

People also refer to IBS as spastic colitis, mucous colitis, and nervous colon. It is a chronic condition. However, its symptoms tend to change over the years. Symptoms often improve as individuals learn to manage the condition.

Until recently, scientists were not sure what caused IBS, but there is growing evidence that microbes present during infectious gastroenteritis may trigger a long-term reaction.

In this article, we discuss symptoms, causes, and treatment, and how diet can affect IBS.

Symptoms

The most common symptoms of IBS include:

- changes in bowel habits

- abdominal pain and cramping, which often reduce after passing a stool

- a feeling that the bowels are not empty after passing stools

- passing excess gas

- the passing of mucus from the rectum

- a sudden, urgent need to use the bathroom

- swelling or bloating of the abdomen

Symptoms often get worse after meals. A flare-up may last for several days, and then symptoms either improve or resolve completely.

Signs and symptoms vary between individuals. They often resemble symptoms of other diseases and conditions and can also affect different parts of the body.

These may include:

- frequent urination

- halitosis, or bad breath

- headache

- joint or muscle pain

- persistent fatigue

- in females, painful sex, or dyspareunia

- irregular menses

Anxiety and depression may also occur, often due to the discomfort and embarrassment that may accompany the condition.

Causes

It is unclear what causes IBS, but experts believe that microbial factors may play a key role.

Scientists have linked it to food poisoning. In fact, 1 in 9 people who experience food poisoning develop IBS at a later date. It seems that the microbes involved in infectious gastroenteritis may have an impact on the immune system that leads to long-term changes in the gut.

Other factors that may play a role include:

- diet

- environmental factors, such as stress

- genetic factors

- hormones

- digestive organs with a high sensitivity to pain

- an unusual response to infection

- a malfunction in the muscles that move food through the body

- an inability of the central nervous system (CNS) to control the digestive system

- A person's mental and emotional state can contribute to IBS development. People with post-traumatic stress disorder (PTSD) have a higher risk of developing IBS.

It is not contagious and does not have links to cancer.

Hormonal changes can make symptoms worse. For example, symptoms are often more severe in women around the time of menstruation.

Infections such as gastroenteritis may trigger post-infectious IBS (PI-IBS).

Is it curable?

There is no cure for IBS. However, if a person with IBS avoids triggers, makes dietary adjustments, and follows their doctor's advice, they can significantly reduce the risk of flares and discomfort.

Treatment options for IBS aim to relieve symptoms and improve quality of life.

Treatment

Treating IBS usually involves some dietary and lifestyle changes, as well as learning how to manage stress.

Dietary management

The following steps may help symptoms:

avoiding sugar alternatives in some chewing gums, diet foods, and sugar free sweets, as they can cause diarrhea

- consuming more oat-based foods to reduce gas or bloating
- not skipping meals
- eating at the same time every day
- eating slowly

- limiting alcohol intake

- avoiding carbonated, sugary beverages, such as soda

- limiting intake of certain fruits and vegetables

- drinking at least 8 cups of fluid per day, for most people

Avoiding gluten can also reduce the risk of flares. Gluten free food products and alternatives are now widely available.

Anxiety and stress

The following may help reduce or relieve symptoms:

- relaxation techniques, including exercises or meditation

- activities such as Tai Chi or yoga

- regular physical exercise

- stress counseling or cognitive-behavioral therapy (CBT)

Medications

The following medications may help IBS symptoms:

- Antispasmodic medications: These reduce abdominal cramping and pain by relaxing the muscles in the gut.

- Bulk-forming laxatives: These can help a person relieve constipation. People should use them with caution.

- Antimotility medications: These can reduce diarrhea symptoms. Options include loperamide, which slows down the contractions of the intestinal muscles.

- Tricyclic antidepressants (TCAs): These often help to reduce abdominal pain and cramping.

Medications specific to IBS treatment include:

- alosetron (Lotronex) for severe diarrhea-predominant IBS in females
- lubiprostone (Amitiza) for constipation-predominant IBS in females
- rifaximin, an antibiotic that can help reduce diarrhea in people with IBS
- eluxadoline

These are usually the last line of treatment when other lifestyle or therapeutic interventions have failed, and symptoms remain severe.

Psychological therapy

Some people may find psychological therapy useful in reducing IBS flares and the impact of symptoms: Techniques include;

- Hypnotherapy: This can help alter the way the unconscious mind responds to physical symptoms.

- Cognitive-behavioral therapy (CBT): This helps people develop strategies for reacting differently to the condition through relaxation techniques and a positive attitude.

Exercise can also help reduce symptoms in some people.

As experts learn more about possible links between IBS and microbial activity there is hope that, one day, new treatments will be available that target this factor effectively.

Diagnosis

Until recently, there was no specific imaging or laboratory test to support an IBS diagnosis. However, experts have now developed a blood test that can accurately reveal whether a person has IBS with diarrhea (IBS-D) or irritable bowel disease (IBD).

During diagnosis, a doctor will aim to rule out conditions that produce symptoms similar to IBS. They will also follow a procedure to categorize the symptoms.

There are three main types of IBS:

- IBS with constipation (IBS-C): A person experiences stomach pain, discomfort, bloating, infrequent or delayed bowel movements, or hard or lumpy stools.

- IBS with diarrhea (IBS-D): There is stomach pain, discomfort, an urgent need to go to the toilet, very frequent bowel movements, or watery or loose stools.

- IBS with alternating stool pattern (IBS-A): A person experiences both constipation and diarrhea.

Many people experience different types of IBS over time. The doctor can often diagnose IBS by asking about symptoms, for example:

- Have there been any changes in bowel habits, such as diarrhea or constipation?

- Is there any pain or discomfort in the abdomen?
- How often does a person feel bloated?

A blood test may help rule out other possible conditions, including:

- lactose intolerance
- small intestinal bacterial overgrowth
- celiac disease

If specific signs or symptoms suggest a different condition, further testing may be necessary. These include:

- anemia
- localized swelling in the rectum and abdomen
- unexplained weight loss

- abdominal pain at night

- progressively worsening symptoms

- significant amounts of blood in the stool

- family history of inflammatory bowel disease (IBD), colorectal cancer, or celiac disease

People with a history of ovarian cancer may require further testing, as might individuals over the age of 60 years with changing bowel habits. This could suggest a risk of bowel cancer.

Risk factors

A 2019 review of 38 studies found that the following characteristics and conditions may increase the risk of IBS:

- gastroenteritis

- being a younger or older adult

- a history of anxiety or depression

- stress

- overusing healthcare

- a family history of IBS

- pain

- sleep disorders

Research into IBS is on-going to develop improved preventive measures and new treatments.

For now, being mindful of diet and stress are the best steps for avoiding flares of discomfort.

Q:

Can I get IBS from eating gluten?

A:

Some people with IBS may have concomitant allergy or sensitivity to gluten. Therefore, ask your doctor to test you for the same.

If you are allergic or sensitive to gluten, then it is a good idea to consider a gluten free diet.

IBS diet

Dietary steps that can help a person reduce the risk of a flare include:

- Managing fiber intake: Some people with IBS need to increase their fiber intake, while others should consume less. A balanced level of fiber in the diet can help promote healthful digestion.

- Probiotic supplements: Taking probiotics may help some people. These are beneficial bacteria that support gut health. A person may not feel their effects immediately, so they should take them over a few weeks to gauge their impact on gut health over a more extended period.

- Food diary: Keeping a record of specific foods in the diet and their physical effects will help a person identify primary trigger foods.

Dietary recommendations for IBS often include the following:

- Eating more soluble fiber: This makes stool easier to pass, while insoluble fiber can aggravate IBS symptoms.

- Eliminating gluten, lactose, or both: Doing so could help ease symptoms.

- Limiting hard-to-digest carbohydrates: Some foods contain high levels of these carbs, which doctors call fermentable oligo-, di-, and monosaccharides and polyols (FODMAPs).

Research indicates that consuming high-FODMAP foods may worsen symptoms of IBS, such as:

- bloating

- stomach pain

- constipation, diarrhea, or both

A doctor or dietitian can help a person make dietary changes aimed at resolving IBS symptoms.

To identify triggers, they may recommend eliminating certain foods, then reintroducing them one by one to check whether each causes symptoms. They may also ask a person to keep a food journal and note when symptoms occur.

Foods that may trigger IBS

Different people may have different food triggers. However, some food groups and specific products are more likely to cause IBS symptoms than others.

The following can trigger symptoms of the syndrome:

- fruits: apples, apricots, blackberries, mangoes, cherries, nectarines, peaches, plums, green bananas, watermelon, and pears, whether whole or in juice

- vegetables: artichokes, cabbage, asparagus, cauliflower, garlic, mushrooms, onions, soybeans, sweetcorn, green peas, snap peas, and snow peas

- pulses: lentils, beans, and chickpeas

- dairy products: milk, ice cream, sour cream, and cottage cheese, unless they are lactose-free

- insoluble fiber: bran, whole grains, nuts, corn, and the skins of fruits and vegetables

- wheat and rye products: breads and other baked goods, as well as products such as sauces that contain wheat flour for thickening

- sweeteners: honey, high fructose corn syrup, and artificial sweeteners, such as sorbitol, maltitol, or xylitol

A person may also want to avoid resistant starches, which are common in whole grains, partially baked breads, and processed foods, such as potato chips.

These reach the large intestine almost undigested, and during digestion in the colon, fermentation occurs, producing gas.

Other products that can cause or worsen IBS symptoms include:

- carbonated drinks

- alcohol

- teas and coffee

- coleslaw

- sauerkraut

- pizza and other greasy foods

- fried foods
- spicy foods
- processed foods
- baked beans
- dishes made from dried pasta
- potato or pasta salads
- pastries
- muesli, which often contains bran

However, keep in mind that the foods and drinks that trigger IBS symptoms vary from person to person. It is important for anyone with this condition to identify their own triggers.

Alternatives to trigger foods

While eliminating foods that cause or worsen IBS symptoms, a person may benefit from adding the following to their diet:

- Low-FODMAP fruits: These include blueberries, cantaloupe, grapes, oranges, kiwis, strawberries, and ripe bananas.

- Low-FODMAP vegetables: These include carrots, eggplant, green beans, spinach, squash, and sweet potatoes.

- Dairy alternatives: Lactose-free products may be a good bet, as may alternatives made from rice, soy, almonds, or oats.

- Yogurt: Some research indicates that probiotics, which can be found in yogurt, may improve IBS symptoms.

- Soluble fiber: Found in oats, psyllium, and some fruits and vegetables, this type of fiber helps regulate bowel movements.

- Sweeteners: Maple syrup without high fructose corn syrup or stevia can be healthful replacements for sweeteners ending in "-ol."

It is also important to focus on healthful fats. For example, try replacing about three-quarters of the butter in a recipe with olive oil. If a recipe calls for 4 tablespoons of butter, try using 3 tablespoons of olive oil and 1 tablespoon of butter.

While it may not be possible to eliminate all the IBS triggers in a recipe, reducing their quantities can help.

The IBS seven-day eating plan

Please note that this eating plan does not replace any advice given by a doctor or nutritionist, and every person who suffers from IBS is different. If for any reason your symptoms worsen, then stop the diet until you have sought further advice.

Day 1

Breakfast Porridge made from 40g quinoa or rice or barley flakes with soya milk, rice milk or water. Serve with a handful of fresh raspberries.

Lunch Half a carton of any fresh soup. 2-3 rice cakes topped with mashed avocado.

Afternoon snack Pot of soya yoghurt, 2 Sesame Snap bars.

Dinner Chicken stir-fried with a little soy sauce, ginger, green peppers and mushrooms. Serve with basmati rice (50-75g dry weight)

Day 2

Breakfast 2-3 rice cakes topped with smooth almond or peanut butter and mashed banana. Glass of oat, rice or soya milk.

Lunch Open sandwich made from sliced pumpernickel or wheat-free rye bread topped with smoked salmon and sliced apple.

Afternoon snack Bowl of any berries served with oat cream or soya yoghurt.

Dinner 2-egg omelette filled with sautéed potato, spinach and red pepper served with steamed broccoli and a dab of red pesto.

Day 3

Breakfast Protein shake made from soya, rice or oat milk with a sachet of whey protein (try Solgar's Whey To Go, £59.25 from health stores or www.solgar.co.uk) mixed with few strawberries.

Lunch Sandwich made from two slices of pumpernickel or rye bread topped with sliced boiled egg, spinach and sliced tomato and a little low fat mayonnaise.

Afternoon snack 2-3 Ryvita or rice cakes topped with smooth nut butter and mashed banana.

Dinner Grilled fillet of any white fish served with ratatouille and mashed sweet potato.

Day 4

Breakfast Cornflakes, Rice Krispies or Special K topped with soya, rice or oat milk. Top with berries.

Lunch Greek-style salad made from chopped lettuce, tomato, olive and feta cheese.

Afternoon snack Piece of rye toast topped with smooth nut butter.

Dinner Grilled chicken breast served with quinoa and roasted vegetables.

Day 5

Breakfast Soya yoghurt served with chopped banana and berries.

Lunch Supermarket rice and vegetable salad served with tinned tuna or crab meat, on a bed of rocket.

Afternoon snack 2-3 rice cakes topped with mashed avocado.

Dinner Lamb chop served with mashed peas and roasted red peppers and courgette.

Day 6

Breakfast Pumpernickel or rye toast topped with poached or scrambled egg.

Lunch Tinned salmon or sardines served with served with low fat supermarket potato salad and unlimited rocket and tomato

Afternoon snack 2 Sesame Snaps and a banana.

Dinner 4-6 scallops pan-fried with a little lemon, served with asparagus and sweet potato mash

Day 7

Breakfast Quinoa or rice porridge, as day one, topped with a pinch of cinnamon and a few sultanas.

Lunch Half a carton of fresh soup served with a slice of rye toast topped with hummus and unlimited salad of rocket, tomato and beetroot

Afternoon snack Bowl of berries served with soya yoghurt or oat cream

Dinner Tuna, salmon or trout fillet, pan-fried. Serve on a bed of spinach with passata drizzled over the top, with 50g (dry weight) of basmati rice

Remember: This diet may not suit everyone, and if you're still experiencing symptoms it's important to see your doctor as soon as possible.

Tips for eating out

Going to a restaurant can be stressful for a person with IBS, but the following strategies can help.

First, be sure to read the menu carefully. Check for ingredients that may cause symptoms and ask:

- What exactly does the dish contain?

- How much of a triggering ingredient is in the dish?

- Is it possible to prepare the dish without the ingredient?

Some people prefer to check the menu online and inquire ahead of time.

Also, it can help to:

Ask for a gluten-free or lactose-free menu: Some restaurants have them.

Check the base of soups: Broth-based soups are less likely to contain cream, which is a trigger for some people.

Find out what vegetable dishes contain: Check the ingredients in a vegetable medley or stir-fry.

Ask about added ingredients: Hamburgers, for example, may contain breadcrumbs or onions, both of which can worsen IBS symptoms.

Opt for grilled (not fried) foods: Grilled foods contain less fat and so can cause less stomach discomfort.

Bring a favorite dressing: Some people take along condiments from home, as commercial dressings and sauces contain additives that aggravate their symptoms.

It may be worth researching a restaurant's options before booking a table.

Other strategies

Many people with IBS find that cooking food at home with fresh ingredients is a good way to avoid symptoms.

Here are some other tips that may help:

- Eat regularly and avoid delaying or missing meals.

- Eat smaller meals.

- Take time when eating.

- Eat no more than 3 servings of fruit a day.

- Limit the intake of tea and coffee to three cups per day.

- Drink plenty of water.

- Eat more protein than carbohydrates.

Outlook

IBS is a common gastrointestinal disorder that can cause significant discomfort. A person's diet can trigger or worsen symptoms.

Identifying and avoiding triggering foods and drinks can help a person with IBS enjoy their meals, at home or during a night out.

IBD DIET RECIPES

In this part are recipes to keep your IBD at bay.

Miso Braised Eggplant

Preparation time

20 minutes

INGREDIENTS

- 2 medium (300g each) eggplants

- 2 tablespoons white miso paste

- 1 tablespoon gluten-free soy sauce

- 2 tablespoons mirin

- 1/2 teaspoon sesame oil

- 2 teaspoons brown sugar

- 2cm piece fresh ginger, peeled, finely grated

- 1 tablespoon vegetable oil

- 1 teaspoon sesame seeds, toasted

- 1 tablespoon chopped fresh chives

- 1 long red chilli, sliced

Instructions

1. Cut each eggplant in half lengthways.

2. Score each cut side in a crisscross pattern.

3. Place miso paste, soy sauce, mirin, sesame oil, sugar, ginger and 1/3 cup water in a small bowl.

4. Stir until smooth.

5. Heat oil in a large, deep frying pan over medium-high heat.

6. Cook eggplant, cut-side down, for 5 minutes or until golden. Turn.

7. Add miso mixture.

8. Reduce heat to medium- low. Cover.

9. Cook for 10 to 12 minutes, turning halfway, or until eggplant is tender.

10. Sprinkle with sesame seeds, chives and chilli.

11. Serve.

Sticky sprout and celeriac mash

Preparation time

20 minutes

INGREDIENTS

- 700g celeriac, peeled, chopped
- 500g desiree potatoes, peeled, coarsely chopped
- 50g butter, chopped
- 150g Brussels sprouts, halved, shredded
- 2 tablespoons maple syrup
- 1/4 cup quark

Instructions

1. Place celeriac and potato in a large saucepan.

2. Cover with cold water.

3. Bring to the boil over medium-high heat.

4. Boil for 15 to 20 minutes or until tender.

5. Meanwhile, melt half the butter in a frying pan over medium-high heat.

6. Add sprouts.

7. Cook, tossing occasionally, for 5 minutes or until just tender.

8. Add half the maple syrup.

9. Cook for 5 minutes or until sprout mixture is golden and sticky.

10. Drain celeriac and potato.

11. Return vegetables to pan.

12. Place pan over low heat for 30 seconds or until excess moisture evaporates.

13. Remove from heat. Using a potato masher, mash vegetables.

14. Add quark and remaining butter.

15. Season with salt and pepper.

16. Beat with a wooden spoon until smooth and creamy.

17. Fold sprout mixture through mash.

18. Serve drizzled with remaining maple syrup.

Coconut Candy

Preparation time

30 minutes

Ingredients

FOR THE BROWNIES

- 350g Medjool dates
- 60g Cocoa powder
- 0.3g (pinch) salt
- ½ Avocado, medium
- 2tsp Vanilla extract
- 100g Coconut flour
- 1tbsp Coconut oil
- 2tbsp Agave

FOR THE ICING

- Coconut cream
- 200ml Coconut cream
- ½ Avocado, medium
- 25g Cocoa powder
- 60g Tapioca flour
- 3tbsp Agave
- 2tsp Vanilla extract

Instructions

1. Line a 9"x5" inch tin with parchment paper and set aside.

2. Strain the coconut cream out, preserving the liquid.

3. Add all of the dough ingredients into a food processor and blend well (approx 2 mins), until mix forms into a breadcrumb-like consistency.

4. Slowly pour the coconut water (strained from the tin) into the mix and blend until a dough forms.

5. Transfer dough into the tin and press firmly, pushing down to get an even consistency throughout the tin. Place in the fridge while preparing the icing.

6. For the icing, add the coconut cream, avocado, cocoa, agave and vanilla extract to the food processor and blitz until smooth (approx 4 mins), stopping to scrape down the sides.

7. Once smooth, slowly start to add the tapioca starch to thicken up the icing. Do one tbsp at a time, until it reaches a thick buttercream consistency.

8. Remove the brownie dough out of the fridge. Spoon the icing on to the brownies and spread out with the back of a spoon until the icing is even.

9. Keep the brownies in a refrigerator until it is time to serve (allow at least 15 mins of chill time.)

10. Carefully remove the brownies from the tin by lifting out the parchment paper and placing it on a chopping board. Cut it into squares of approx 1.5"-2".

11. Serve and enjoy!

Greek Lamb Salad

Preparation time

30 minutes

Ingredients

- 400gms/14 oz lamb steak

- 1 tsp dried thyme

- Zest of ½ a lemon

- Salt and pepper

- 2 big tomatoes

- ½ cup black olives

- Mint

- A packet of rocket

- 4 tbsp pesto (homemade with garlic-infused oil)

- 2 tbsp lemon juice

- 1 tbsp olive oil

- 2 red bell peppers

- 150gms/5.3oz feta

Instructions

1. Rub the lemon zest, thyme, salt and pepper into the steaks.

2. Place on a hot grill and cook to seal on the outside but take off with the meat pink on the inside.

3. Rest 10 minutes.

4. Slice into ½"/1.25cm thick pieces

5. Place the two peppers on an open flame and keep turning to blacken all the skin.

6. Cool and rub off the skin.

Slice into strips.

7. Slice up the tomatoes.

8. Rip the mint into pieces.

9. Cut the feta into cubes.

10. Place all the ingredients into a serving bowl or layer on a big platter.

11. Combine the pesto, lemon juice and olive oil to make a dressing.

12. Drizzle the dressing over the platter or toss the salad in the bowl to combine all ingredients with the dressing.

Blueberry And Lemon Buttermilk Pancakes

Preparation time

30 minutes

Ingredients

- 300ml lactose free or almond mil

- 1 tablespoon lemon juice

- 200g gluten free plain flour
- 50g rolled oats, gluten free if needed
- 1 1/2 teaspoons baking powder
- 1/2 teaspoon baking soda
- 1/2 teaspoon salt
- 1 tablespoon brown sugar
- Zest of 1/2 a lemon
- 1 Clarence Court Leghorn Whites free range egg
- 25g butter, melted, plus extra for frying
- 150g blueberries
- Maple syrup

Instructions

1. First make the 'buttermilk' by combining the almond milk and 1 tablespoon lemon juice and whisk together.

2. Let sit for 5-7 minutes to 'curdle'.

3. Mix together the flour, oats, baking powder, baking soda, salt, sugar and lemon zest in a large bowl.

4. Beat the egg with the milk, make a well in the centre of the dry ingredients and whisk in the milk to make a thick batter.

5. Beat in the melted butter and place the batter back in the fridge for ten minutes to rest (and to let the gluten free flour soak up all that liquid).

6. Heat a small knob of butter in a large non-stick frying pan.

7. Drop two large tablespoonful of the batter per pancake into the pan.

8. Scatter the batter with blueberries.

9. Cook for about 3 minutes over a medium heat until small bubbles appear on the surface of each pancake, then turn and cook another 2-3 minutes until golden.

10. Cover with a clean kitchen towel to keep warm while you use up the rest of the batter.

Muesli

Preparation time

30 minutes

Ingredients

- 250 g (5 cups) gluten free cornflakes*
- 38 g (1 1/2 cup) quinoa puffs*
- 7 tbsp dried shredded coconut*
- 4 tbsp pumpkin seeds*
- 65 g (1/3 cup)   brown sugar
- 6 tbsp olive oil
- 30 g dried banana chips (15 chips)*

Equipment

- roasting dish

Instructions

1. Preheat the oven to 150ºC or 300ºF on bake function.

2. Measure out the cornflakes and roughly crush them (I did this by putting them in a plastic bag and then crushing them with a rolling pin).

3. In a large bowl mix the cornflakes, quinoa puffs, dried shredded coconut, pumpkin seeds and brown sugar.

4. Add the oil and mix through the muesli until it is evenly covered.

5. Line an oven roasting tray with baking paper.

6. Add the muesli evenly to the tray.

7. Place in the oven and allow to toast, tossing every 10 minutes until light brown (should take 15 to 20 minutes).

8. Remove from oven and allow to cool.

9. Lightly crush the banana chips and add to the muesli.

10. Transfer the muesli to an air tight container or jar.

11. You can store it for up to two weeks.

12. Serve

Kiwi Smoothie

Preparation time

5 minutes

INGREDIENTS:

- 1 cup (170 g) seedless green grapes

- 1 kiwi, peeled and cut into chunks

- 2 tablespoons water

- 8- inches (20 cm) of unpeeled English, hothouse style cucumber, cut into chunks

- 2 cups (40 g) baby spinach, (for a milder taste) or chopped stemmed, washed and dried

Lacinato kale leaves (for a bolder taste) or a combo

- 1 ½ to 2 cups ice cubes

Instructions

1. Place all the items in blender in order listed - except the ice.

2. Pulse on an off to begin blending, then blend on high speed until puréed, blended and smooth. Add the smaller amount of ice cubes and blend until frosty, pulsing on and off.

3. Add more ice cubes if desired.

4. Serve immediately.

Chocolate Chip-Oat Scones

Preparation time

40 minutes

INGREDIENTS

- 60 g rolled ("Old Fashioned") oats (1/2 cup plus 2 tbsp)

- 100 g King Arthur multi-purpose gluten-free flour blend (1/2 cup plus 2 tbsp), plus additional for rolling dough

- 2 1/2 tbsp granulated sugar

- 1 1/4 tsp baking powder

- 1/4 tsp xanthan gum

- 1/4 tsp salt

- 1 large or extra large egg (works with whatever size you keep on hand)

- 2 tbsp lactose-free milk or lactose-free yogurt

- 2 tsp vanilla extract

- 57 g cold unsalted butter, cut into small cubes (4 tbsp)

- 65 g mini dark chocolate chips (see note above) (1/4 cup)

Instructions

1. Preheat oven to 350F.

2. Spread oats on a large rimmed baking sheet (I use a light-colored baking sheet.

3. If you have a dark baking sheet, consider reducing oven temp to 375F or checking a couple minutes early to avoid over-browning the bottoms of the scones) and bake until lightly toasted, stirring once with a spatula, 5 to 6 minutes.

4. Raise oven temp to 400F and measure out a piece of parchment paper that you'll use to line the same baking sheet for the scones.

5. In a large bowl, whisk together the flour, sugar, baking powder, xanthan gum and salt. In a medium bowl, whisk together the egg, milk or yogurt and vanilla; set aside.

6. Add the cold butter to the flour mixture.

7. Using a pastry blender (or a fork, or your fingertips), work the butter into the flour until

you have a coarse, sandy mixture with chunks the size of small peas.

8. Stir in the oats. Add the egg mixture and raisins and stir just until dry ingredients are moistened.

9. Sprinkle a cutting board or work surface generously with flour and scoop the dough onto the flour.

10. With floured hands, knead dough into a ball. If a good amount of dry crumbs of dough still remain, drizzle with a few drops of additional milk or yogurt to help incorporate them (be super-conservative, as it is very easy to over-hydrate gluten-free dough).

11. Press the dough into a thick disk and use a rolling pin to roll into a circle, about 3/4-inch thick.

12. Dust the dough and rolling pin with flour to prevent sticking.

13. Cut dough into 6 wedges.

14. Line the baking sheet with the parchment paper and transfer the wedges to the baking sheet, leaving a few inches of space between them.

15. Bake in the center of the oven until edges are light golden brown and a toothpick comes out clean, 12 to 14 minutes (rotate the baking sheet after about 8 minutes for even baking). Rest on baking sheet 3 to 5 minutes, then

transfer to a wire rack. These are great warm or at room temp and they freeze VERY well.

16. Defrost at room temp for 30 minutes to an hour, and they taste perfect and fresh.

COCONUT OAT GRANOLA WITH CHOCOLATE AND ROSEWATER CREAM

Preparation time

40 minutes

Ingredients

- 90g oats, blended into flour (certified gluten free if needed)

- 90g shredded coconut

- 80ml coconut oil, liquid

- 60ml maple syrup

- 1/8 tsp sea salt

- 1 tin (400ml) full-fat coconut milk (left in the fridge overnight)

- 1 tsp rosewater

- 1 tsp vanilla extract

- 100g dark chocolate, broken into pieces

- Almond or other milk, to serve

- Edible flowers or fresh fruit

Instructions

1. Preheat oven to 180ºC/350ºF/Gas Mark 4.

2. To make the crust, combine coconut oil, maple syrup, oat flour and shredded coconut together in a mixing bowl.

3. Grease a small baking tin with coconut oil and press mixture into the bottom before placing into the oven and cook for 15-20 minutes until crispy.

4. Remove from the oven and set aside to cool and firm up.

5. Meanwhile, scoop out the solid coconut cream from the tin and into a large bowl.

6. Stop scooping when you reach the water in the bottom of the can (save this for smoothies later).

7. Using a mixer or hand beaters on high speed - whip the coconut cream for 3 to 5 minutes until it becomes fluffy and light, with soft peaks.

8. Stir through the vanilla and rosewater.

9. Once the granola has cooked and cooled, break up into chunks and divide across bowls.

10. Top with rosewater cream, dark chocolate and edible flowers or fresh fruit.

11. Serve with your favourite lactose- or dairy-free milk.

POACHED EGG WITH YOGURT AND GARLIC-INFUSED OIL

Preparation time

10 minutes

Ingredients

- large organic egg

- 1 Tbsp garlic-infused olive oil, store-bought (e.g. this one) or homemade

- 1 pinch chili flakes

- 1/8 tsp dried paprika powder

- 150 grams (approx. 1 cup) greek style yogurt (use lactose free if necessary)
- 1 pinch of sea salt

Instructions

1. Add the egg to a pot of simmering water and cook for 5 minutes.

2. It should still be runny inside.

3. In a small saucepan or pan, slowly heat garlic-infused oil, chili flakes and paprika powder.

4. Take off from heat and allow to infuse until the egg is ready.

5. Add the yogurt to a small bowl, peel the egg and place on top of the yogurt.

6. Pour infused oil over the egg and sprinkle with sea salt.

7. Serve immediately and enjoy with bread and veggies of your choice.

Note

- Serve with: Fresh spelt bread, warm corn tortilla or pita bread, fresh sprouts and veggies

Quinoa Porridge with Berries

Preparation time

30 minutes

Ingredients

- 85 g (1/2 cup) quinoa*

- 1 tsp neutral oil (rice bran, canola, sunflower)

- 250 ml (1 cup) water

- 188 ml (3/4 cup) low FODMAP milk*

- 1/4 tsp ground cinnamon*

- 4 tsp pure maple syrup*

- 10 raspberries (fresh or frozen)

- 20 blueberries (fresh or frozen)

Instructions

1. Measure out the quinoa.

2. Using a fine mesh sieve rinse it under cold running water for two minutes.

3. Transfer it to a medium sized saucepan and add a drizzle of neutral oil.

4. Toast the quinoa over medium heat for 1 to 2 minutes until the water has evaporated and the quinoa is lightly toasted.

5. Add the water.

6. Bring the quinoa to a rolling boil and then turn down the element to the lowest heat setting. Cover with a pot lid and allow to cook for 12 to 15 minutes.

7. The quinoa should be quite fluffy.

8. Drain off any excess water if needed and return to pan.

9. Then add the low FODMAP milk, cinnamon, and maple syrup.

10. Then allow the porridge to simmer for about 5 minutes or until heated through.

11. If you are using frozen berries and want them heated then add them to the mixture.

12. Serve the hot quinoa porridge into bowls and divide the raspberries and blueberries equally between them.

Spaghetti Bolognese

Preparation time

40 minutes

Ingredients

- 1 tbsp olive oil
- 500g lean ground beef
- 40 g (1/2 cup) leek (green tips only)*
- 400 g plain crushed/chopped tomatoes (canned)*
- 3 tbsp tomato paste
- 1 tsp dried oregano*
- 1 tsp dried basil*
- 1/2 tsp dried thyme*
- 120 g (4 cups) baby spinach
- Season with salt & pepper (to taste)
- 300 g gluten free spaghetti*

- 57 g (1/2 cup) colby or cheddar cheese or vegan cheese (optional) (grated)*

Instructions

1. Roughly chop the baby spinach and finely chop the green leek tips.

2. Peel and cut the carrots into sticks and slice the green beans into bite sized pieces.

3. Place to one side.

4. Select a large fry pan and place on medium heat.

5. Add a splash of olive oil and cook lean ground beef until browned.

6. Add the canned tomatoes, tomato paste, leek tips, baby spinach and herbs (oregano, basil, thyme) to the lean ground beef.

7. Mix well and allow to simmer on medium to low heat for 20 minutes. Make sure you stir it so it doesn't burn.

8. Add salt and pepper to taste.

9. Add a generous amount of salt to a large saucepan of water.

10. Bring the water to a rolling boil.

11. Then add the gluten free spaghetti and cook according to packet directions, until soft.

12. Drain pasta and toss with olive oil.

13. While the spaghetti cooks, cook the green beans and carrots in a medium sized saucepan

of boiling water for two to three minutes, until they are brightly coloured and soft.

14. Serve the bolognese on top of spaghetti and sprinkle with a low FODMAP cheese like cheddar or colby (if desired).

15. Make sure you include the veggies on the side (I like to mix mine in with the bolognese).

Maple Garlic Glazed Salmon

Preparation time

50 minutes

Ingredients

- Serves 2-3 people

- 1/2 pound salmon filet

- 2 tablespoons pure maple syrup

- 1 tablespoon garlic infused oil

- 1 tablespoon soy sauce

- Salt and pepper, to taste

- Dash of either crushed red pepper or sesame seeds

Instructions

1. Preheat oven to 400 degrees F

2. In small bowl mix maple syrup, soy sauce, garlic infused oil, salt, and pepper

3. Place salmon in small glass baking dish and coat with maple and garlic infused mixture.

4. Marinate in refrigerator for 25-30 minutes.

5. Sprinkle with crushed red pepper flakes or sesame seeds, as desired

6. Bake uncovered in oven for 20 minutes or until flaky and cooked through.

Bibimbap Nourishing Bowl

Preparation time

50 minutes

Ingredients

- ½ cup brown rice
- 1 cup water
- Pinch of salt

- 2 cups | 2,65oz | 75g swiss chard without stems OR spinach chopped

- 2,65 oz | 75g rainbow carrot peeled and julienned

- 2,29 oz | 65g courgette julienned

- 3 tbsp olive oil

- 6 oz | 170g plain tofu

- Pinch of salt

- 2 eggs (optional. Omit if vegetarian)

- 0,56 oz | 4g green onions green tops only, chopped

- 1 tbsp | 0,39oz | 11g Sesame seeds (optional)

Instructions

1. Place the rice in a sauce pan with boiling water and a pinch of salt.

2. Cook on a low heat, until all the water has been absorbed and the rice is cooked.

3. Drain and wrap the tofu with paper towel.

4. Place a plate and a heavy object on top of the tofu and set aside for 15 minutes. This process will help tofu drain faster.

5. After pressing the tofu, cut into medium rectangular strips and coat both sides with salt.

6. In a hot grill pan, grill 5 minutes per side or until crispy and golden brown.

7. For the swiss chard, carrots and zucchini, simply heat up 2 tbsp of olive oil in a skillet, then

sauté the vegetables (one at a time) with salt until tender.

8. Chard will take 5-7 minutes, carrots about 5 minutes, and zucchini 2-4 minutes.

9. Fry the eggs (optional) with a tbsp of olive oil and add a pinch of salt.

10. Place the rice in two bowls, top with veggies and tofu, and finish with a sunny side up egg.

11. Top with green onions and sesame seeds (optional), stir everything up and serve.

Chilli Coconut Crusted Fish with Salad

Preparation time

45 minutes

Ingredients

- Chilli Coconut Crust

- 20 g (1/4 cup)   dried shredded coconut*

- 2 tbsp   sesame oil

- 10 g (1/4 cup)   green onions/scallions (green tips only, finely sliced)*

- 1   mild green chilli (finely sliced)

- 4   makrut (kaffir) lime leaves (Or lime zest) (fresh, finely sliced)*

- 460 g   mild white fleshed fish (Cod, Haddock, Coley, Pollack, Red Snapper)

- 57 g (1/2 cup)   colby or cheddar cheese or vegan cheese (optional) (grated)*

Homemade Chips

- 700 g potatoes
- Season with salt & pepper
- 1 tbsp neutral oil (rice bran, canola, sunflower)

Salad

- 1 small cucumber (peeled)
- 4 cups lettuce (butter, iceberg, red coral) (washed & shredded)
- 0.5 red bell pepper (deseeded & sliced into strips)
- 4 medium tomatoes (cut into wedges)

- 1 lemon

Equipment

- large frypan

Ingredients

1. To make the chilli coconut crust, place the shredded coconut in a small bowl and cover with water. Leave to soak for 10 minutes before draining. De-seed the mild green chillies and finely slice. Finely slice the green part of the green onions/scallions and the kaffir lime leaves. Add half the sesame oil into a large fry pan and over medium/high heat and fry the green onions/scallions, chilli, and kaffir lime leaves

until golden and fragrant (should look caramelised). Add the drained coconut and fry for another minute. Then set aside and keep for later.

2. In the same large fry pan add the remaining oil and add half the potatoes. Fry until golden and cooked. Then repeat with the second half of the potatoes. Season the fries with salt and black pepper.

3. Prepare the salad ingredients and squeeze the lemon juice over top.

4. Spray a medium sized frying pan with oil and cook the fish for 2 minutes before flipping and cooking for a further 1 or 2 minutes until cooked through. Place the fish on a baking tray, top with grated cheese and cover with the chilli coconut

crust. Grill/broil in the oven on high for 1 to 2 minutes until the crust turns golden.

5. Serve with potato chips and salad

LASAGNA BOLOGNESE

Preparation time

60 minutes

INGREDIENTS

- 350 g minced meat

- 500 ml sieved tomatoes

- 1 paprika

- 100 g carrots

- 150 g canned mushrooms*

- 1 tsp Italian herbs

- 9 – 10 gluten-free lasagna noodles

- 100 g grated cheese

FOR THE BECHAMEL SAUCE

- 25 g butter

- 25 g gluten-free flour

- 300 ml lactose-free milk

- Pepper and salt

Instructions

1. Pre-heat the oven to 175 degrees Celsius.

2. Cut the carrot and the paprika into small pieces. Rinse the mushrooms and drain well.

3. Fry the minced meat until done. Add the vegetables and bake for a few minutes.

4. Add the sieved tomatoes and the Italian herbs and season the sauce with pepper and salt.

5. Make the bechamel sauce by melting the butter in a pan on low heat. Add, when the butter has melted, the flour and stir for 2 minutes with a whisk.

6. Add the milk little by little. Continue to stir with the whisk, so you get a smooth sauce.

7. Stir 30 g of the grated cheese into the bechamel sauce and season with salt and pepper. Leave the sauce to boil on low heat for a few minutes, so it can thicken.

8. Take your oven dish. Put a thin layer of tomato sauce into the oven dish. Then a layer of lasagna noodles and then a layer of bechamel sauce. Continue with tomato sauce and another layer of lasagna noodles. Repeat this until you have used all noodles. I made three layers using 3 lasagna noodles at a time. End with a layer of tomato sauce and divide the rest of the cheese over the top of the lasagna.

9. Bake the lasagna in the oven for 40 minutes. Cover the oven dish with aluminium foil after 20 minutes, otherwise the top of the lasagna might burn.

NOTES

- Normal mushrooms are high in FODMAPs, but canned mushrooms are low FODMAP up to 110 g per portion.

Cheesy Baked Quinoa and Zucchini Cups

Preparation time

35 minutes

Ingredients

- 1/2 cup cooked quinoa
- 1/2 cup grated zucchini
- 1/2 cup grated cheese

- 6 beaten eggs

Instructions

1. Combine all ingredients, mix well, and pour into individual patty cake cases which have been placed in a muffin tray.

2. Bake in the oven 180 degrees Celsius for 20 minutes.

Banana Nut Quinoa Muffins

Preparation time

30 minutes

Ingredients:

Dry Ingredients

- 1 & 1/2 C quinoa flour
- 1 C quinoa flakes
- 1/3 C walnuts or pecans, chopped
- 1 Tbsp. cinnamon
- 4 tsp. baking powder
- 2 tsp. baking soda
- 1 tsp. salt

Wet Ingredients

- 4 flax eggs (or 4 real eggs)
- 4 very ripe bananas, mashed
- 1/2 cup almondmilk

- 1/4 C maple syrup

Instructions:

1. Preheat your oven to 350 degrees F.

2. First, prepare your flax eggs and place them in the fridge to gel.

3. Then, in a large bowl, mix all dry ingredients.

4. In a separate smaller bowl, mix mashed bananas, almondmilk, and maple syrup, then mix in gelled flax eggs.

5. Add wet ingredients to dry ingredients and stir until more or less uniform.

6. Spoon batter into greased muffin pans; place in the oven for 20 minutes.

7. Fork check to test done-ness.

8. Enjoy!

Kettle Popcorn Recipe; Gluten-free, Vegan

Preparation time

5 minutes

Ingredients

- 1/2 cup vegetable oil
- 1 cup popcorn kernels
- 2/3 cup sugar

- 2 teaspoon salt (alter based on your preference)

Instructions

1. Heat the oil in a large pot over medium-high heat

2. Put one kernel in the pot.

3. When it pops, the oil is hot enough

4. Add the popcorn and sugar.

5. Give the kernels a quick stir and then cover with a lid

6. I usually put on oven mitts and the whole time I swirl the pot on the burner so the kernels get evenly heated and don't burn

7. Once the popping slows down, remove immediately from the heat and pour the kettle corn into a large bowl

8. If you don't take it off the heat it will burn the sugar

9. Sprinkle with salt and serve immediately

Homemade Trail mix

Preparation time

5 minutes

Ingredients

- 1 cup pretzel sticks (FODMAP followers use Snyders gluten free pretzels)

- 1/4 cup pumpkin seeds

- 1/4 cup dark or semi-sweet chocolate chips

- 1/2 cup banana chips

Instructions

1. Mix and store in mason jar and enjoy as desired.

Chewy Peanut Butter Cookies

Ingredients

- Makes about 16 cookies

- 1 cup all natural peanut butter (stir well)

- 1/2 cup granulated sugar

- 1 egg

- 1/2 cup gluten free oat flour

- 1 teaspoon baking soda

- Option: Add in 1/4 cup of semi-sweet chocolate chips and/or chopped peanut

Instructions

1. Preheat oven to 350 degrees F.

2. Line cookie sheet with parchment paper

3. Mix together peanut butter, sugar, egg in medium bowl with a spoon until creamy.

4. Blend in flour and baking soda.

5. Fold in chocolate chips and/or nuts if using.

6. Scoop out by tablespoon onto cookie sheet leaving about 1 1/2 inch between cookies.

7. Bake for 8-10 minutes (cookies should be lightly brown on edges)

Blueberry Crumble Slice

Preparation time

60 minutes

Ingredients

Crumble Base

- 156 g (3/4 cup) white sugar
- 420 g (3 cups) gluten free self raising flour*

- 1/4 tsp salt

- 1/2 tsp ground cinnamon*

- 1 tsp guar gum (or xanthan gum) (optional)*

- 250 g dairy free spread (olive oil spread or butter)*

- 1 large egg

Crumble Filling

- 52 g (1/4 cup) white sugar

- 445 g (3 cups) blueberries (fresh or frozen)

- 3 tsp corn starch*

Equipment

- baking tin 20cm by 30cm (12 inch by 8 inch)

Instructions

1. Preheat the oven to 180°C (350°F) bake function.

2. Grease a 20 x 30cm (7.9 inch by 11.8 inch) baking pan. If you want you can line the pan with baking paper.

3. Place 3/4 cup of sugar, 3 cups of gluten free self rising flour, salt and ground cinnamon into a medium sized bowl.

4. Mix well. If using guar gum (or xantham) then add it now. The gum will help the mixture be less crumbly but you don't have to use it.

5. Mix the gum through the dry ingredients.

6. Lightly beat the egg in a small bowl.

7. Place the dairy free spread (olive oil spread or butter) in a bowl and soften slightly in the microwave (you want it soft to touch but not melted).

8. Pour the soft dairy free spread spread and the egg into the dry ingredients.

9. Blend using a fork until the wet ingredients have absorbed into the dry ingredients.

10. Then rub the mixture between your fingers until it turns into quite large moist crumbs.

11. Pat half of the mixture into the pan. It needs to be pressed in firmly until the dough forms a smooth layer.

12. Add the blueberries evenly to the baking pan until they cover the dough.

13. In a small bowl mix together the 3 teaspoons of corn starch and 1/4 cup of sugar.

14. Then evenly sprinkle the sugar mixture on top.

15. Crumble the remaining dough over the blueberry mixture.

16. Bake in the oven for 30 minutes or until top is slightly golden.

17. Let the slice cool before cutting it into 15 pieces.

18. Serve warm with a side of low FODMAP icecream.

19. Remember to only have 1 piece in a sitting.

This slice also freezes well.

Fudgy One-Bowl Brownies

Preparation time

47 minutes

INGREDIENTS

- 250 grams (1 1/4 cups) granulated sugar

- 140 g (10 tbsp) unsalted butter

- 65 g (2/3 cup) Dutch process or "dark" cocoa powder

- 1 tsp instant espresso powder (optional)

- 1/2 tsp sea salt

- 1 tsp vanilla extract

- 2 cold large eggs

- 65 g (1/4 cup plus 2 1/2 tbsp) gluten free flour blend with no gums, such as King Arthur Multi Purpose

- 125 to 140g (2/3 to 3/4 cup) dark chocolate chips/chunks (optional)

INSTRUCTIONS

1. Preheat oven to 350F. Line 8 x 8-inch baking pan (I used a light-colored metal pan) with nonstick foil or parchment paper, leaving an overhang on 2 opposite sides.

2. In a large, microwave-safe bowl, combine the sugar, butter, cocoa, espresso powder if using, and salt.

3. Microwave in 20 to 30-second bursts, stirring each time, until butter is melted. Stir until combined (mixture will be very grainy).

4. Stir in the vanilla.

5. Add the eggs one at a time, stirring until combined after each one.

6. Stir until the batter is thick and shiny.

7. Add the flour and stir until thoroughly combined and no white streaks remain. Stir in chips if using.

8. Spread evenly in prepared pan.

9. Bake until a toothpick comes out with a moist crumbs, 30 to 34 minutes (mine took 32).

10. The top should be puffed and shiny and the brownies pulling away from the sides of the pan.

11. Cool completely on a wire rack.

12. Cut into 12 or 16 brownies.

13. For a perfectly clean cut, put the cooled brownies into the refrigerator or freezer until cold (don't freeze completely). For storage, these freeze really well.

14. You can wrap individual brownies in plastic wrap and store in a ziploc bag. Defrost at room temperature.

Creamy Coconut Milk Quinoa Pudding

Preparation time

50 minutes

Ingredients

- 3/4 cup uncooked quinoa (red, white, tri-color), drain and rinse

- 1 (14 ounce) can light coconut milk

- 2 Tablespoons 100% pure maple syrup

- 1 teaspoon vanilla extract or vanilla bean paste

- Garnish: 1 Tablespoon whipped cream and fresh blueberries

Instructions

1. Bring coconut milk and quinoa in small sauce pan to boil over high heat.

2. Reduce heat to medium low, add in maple syrup and vanilla and continue to cook, stirring occasionally, about 30 minutes until mixture is creamy and pudding light consistency.

3. Place mixture in bowl in refrigerator to cool down, a couple hours.

4. Serve about 1/2 -3/4 cup serving of pudding in small dish.

5. Garnish with a dollop of whipped cream and handful of fresh blueberries.

6. Add some almond slices or walnuts if desired, 1 Tablespoon, chopped.

FERRERO ROCHER

Preparation time

60 minutes

Ingredients

- 100g roasted hazelnuts

- 100g walnuts

- 3 tbsp cacao or cocoa powder

- 2 tbsp coconut oil, melted

- 2 tbsp maple syrup

- 1 tsp pure vanilla extract

- 1/2 tsp sea salt

- Chopped hazelnuts (to garnish)

Instructions

1. Set aside roughly 20 hazelnuts for the centres of the Ferrero Rocher.

2. Add the rest of the hazelnuts and walnuts into a food processor and blend until chopped into small pieces.

3. Add the cacao and sea salt and blend again.

4. Add the maple syrup, vanilla extract and coconut oil and blend until the ingredients start to stick together (you might have to scrape

down the sides of your processor every so often).

5. Roll the mixture into small balls and pop insert a hazelnut in the centre of each one.

6. Cover the outside in chopped hazelnuts.

7. Place the balls in the freezer for 20-30 minutes to harden and store in the fridge.

SOMMER'S STROGANOFF

Preparation time

25 minutes

INGREDIENTS

Nutrition

1 1/4 lbs lean ground turkey (the leaner, the better)

1/2 teaspoon salt

1/4 teaspoon black pepper

1/2 - 3/4 cup chopped white onion

1 tablespoon garlic powder

2 cups sliced white mushrooms (I used the presliced white mushrooms bought from the produce section)

12 ounces uncooked pasta (usually stroganoff is made with egg noodles. I have to use No Yolks. They come in 8oz packages)

24 ounces creamy portabella mushroom soup (Imagine is a brand of non-dairy cream of soup substitute)

1 tablespoon tofutti better-than-cream-cheese (or other subsitutute, I recommend Tofutti brand Better Than

Instructions

1. Brown the ground turkey with the onion, garlic powder, salt, and pepper until meat is completely done.

2. Drain and set aside in a small bowl.

3. Meanwhile, saute the sliced mushrooms in as little margarine as necessary.

4. Cook the No Yolks per package directions in a large pot, except cook them until al dente.

5. When the mushrooms are done, set them aside wrapped in a double layer of paper towels in a bowl to absorb any extra margarine.

6. Drain the No Yolks and rinse with hot water as directed on the package.

7. In the large pot used to boil the noodles in, add the browned ground turkey mixture, sauteed mushrooms, drained noodles, the Tofutti Better Than Cream Cheese, and the soup.

8. Mix well and heat on high to a gentle boil, stirring often.

9. Serve immediately.

Baked French Toast

Preparation time

9 hours

Ingredients

- 1 full COBS LowFOD™ Loaf cut into cubes
- 7 eggs beaten
- 2 cups unsweetened almond milk
- ½ tsp cinnamon
- 2 tsp vanilla extract
- 2 tsp maple syrup
- Pinch salt

- ¼ cup chopped natural peanuts

- Chia Jam:

- 3 cups frozen strawberries or raspberries

- 3 tbsp chia seeds

- 2 tbsp lemon juice

- 2 tsp maple syrup

- 1/3 cup natural peanut butter plus more for drizzling if desired

Topping:

- 2 tbsp melted butter

- 2 tbsp maple syrup

- 2 tbsp brown sugar

Instructions

1. In a 9" square baking dish, mix together the eggs, almond milk, cinnamon, vanilla, salt and maple syrup.

2. Add the chopped COBS LowFOD™ Loaf and allow to sit in the fridge overnight.

3. Meanwhile, heat the frozen berries in a small saucepot along with the lemon juice and maple syrup.

4. Mash the berries until jammy, then take off the heat.

5. Add the chia seeds and allow to sit for 1 hour or more in the fridge to thicken.

6. The next day, preheat oven to 350°

7. Mix the chopped peanuts into the bread and add about 1/3 cup of the chia jam and peanut butter in dollops, pushing it down into the bread casserole.

8. Mix together the topping ingredients of melted butter, maple syrup and brown sugar and drizzle on top of the casserole.

9. Bake for 45-60 minutes or until golden brown and bubbly.

10. Serve with additional chia jam and peanut butter drizzle.

PALEO & LOW FODMAP SWEET AND SOUR CHICKEN

Preparation time

30 minutes

INGREDIENTS

- 1 pound boneless, skinless chicken breasts, cut into 1-inch chunks
- 1/2 cup (65 grams) arrowroot starch or cornstarch
- 1 large egg beaten
- 2 tablespoons coconut oil
- 1/2 cup (100 gram) coconut sugar or regular white sugar
- 1/4 cup (60ml) apple cider vinegar*

- 2 tablespoons Coconut Aminos, or gluten free soy sauce/tamari

- 1/4 cup (60 g) ketchup or Low FODMAP Ketchup

- 1/4 cup (60 ml) chicken stock

- 1 red pepper cut into chunks

- 1 cup (65 g) pineapple chunks

- 3 spring onions stalks, green part only for low fodmap

INSTRUCTIONS

1. First prepare the sauce by adding the coconut sugar, vinegar, coconut aminos, chicken stock and ketchup to a medium sauce pan.

2. Stir and bring to a boil.

3. Reduce to a low heat and leave until later.

4. Add chicken pieces and beaten egg to a large ziplock bag.

5. Seal and shake to coat chicken.

6. Then add the arrowroot starch to the bag, shaking again to lightly coat all the chicken pieces.

7. Add coconut oil to a large non skillet.

8. Add the coated chicken.

9. Fry over medium heat, a couple of minutes on each side until the coating begins to crisp. Add pepper and pineapple chunks.

10. Continue to saute over medium heat until chicken is browned and cooked through.

11. Add the sauce to chicken and peppers.

12. Cover and reduce the heat down to a simmer and allow the juices to soak into the chicken for a few minutes.

13. Top with sliced green onions.

14. Serve over rice and enjoy!

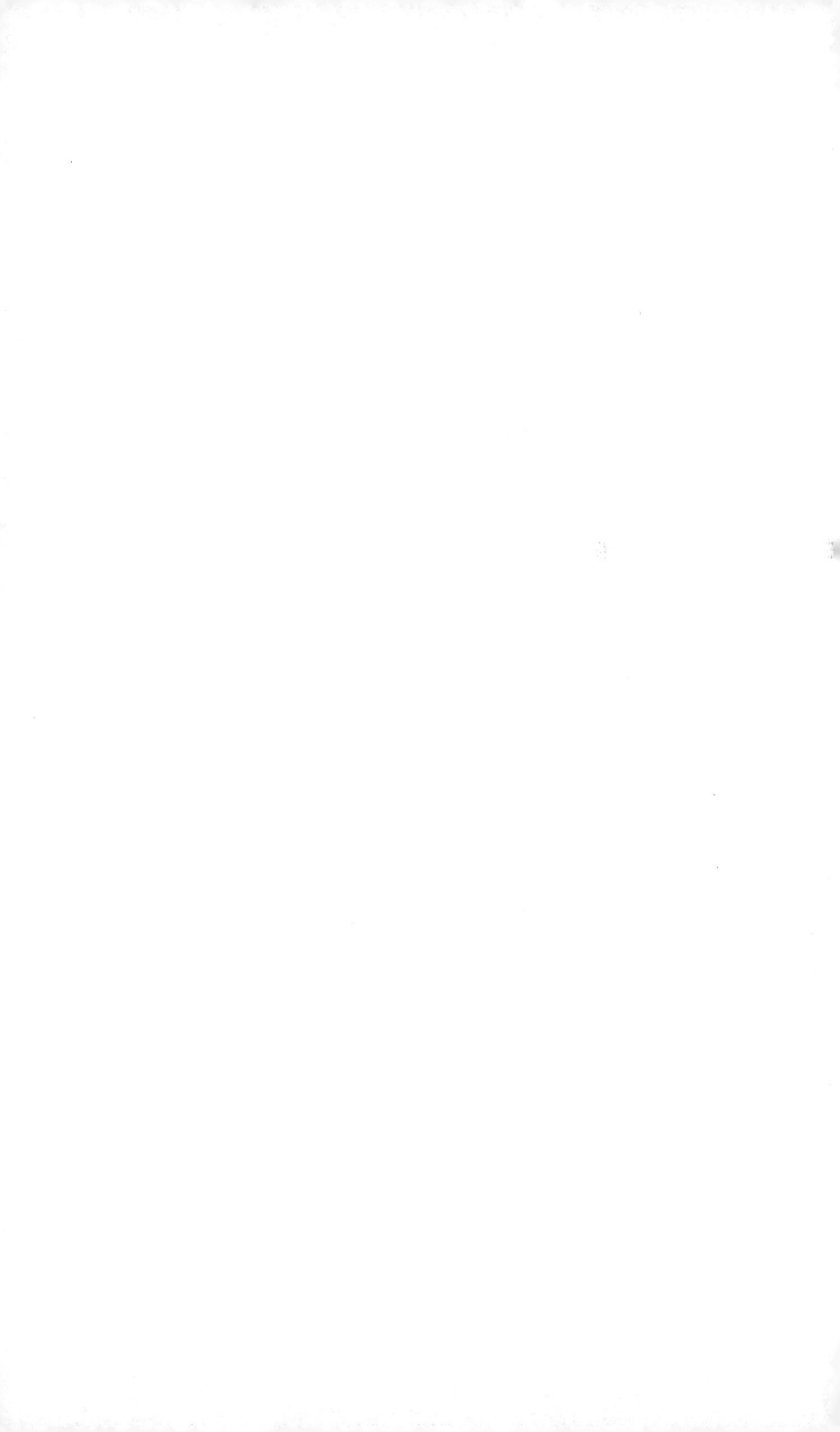

Printed in Great Britain
by Amazon